Application of NLP in Health Coaching:

Improving Patient Compliance and Health Outcomes

By Rex Morton

Copyright Page

© 2023 by Rex Morton

This book is a work of non-fiction. Unless otherwise noted, the author and the publisher make no explicit guarantees as to the accuracy of the information contained in this book and will not be held responsible for any errors or omissions.

Published by Omniterra Media Inc

First Edition

Visit the author's website at www.rexmorton.com

For information regarding special discounts for bulk purchases, please contact Rex Morton @ Rex@rexmorton.com.

Disclaimer

This book is intended to provide information about the fields of Neuro-Linguistic Programming (NLP) and Cognitive Behavioural Therapy (CBT) and their potential integration. While the author has made every effort to ensure that the information was correct at the time of publication, the author does not assume and hereby disclaims any liability to any party for any loss, damage, or disruption caused by errors or omissions, whether such errors or omissions result from negligence, accident, or any other cause.

The contents of this book should not be used as a substitute for professional advice, diagnosis, or treatment. The reader should always consult with a qualified healthcare provider about any mental health concerns or conditions. Never disregard professional psychological or medical advice or delay in seeking it because of something you have read in this book.

The views expressed in this work are solely those of the author and do not necessarily reflect the views of the publisher, and the publisher hereby disclaims any responsibility for them.

The inclusion of websites, links, or references to other resources does not mean that the author or the publisher endorses the information the organization or website may provide or recommendations it might make. Furthermore, the author does not guarantee the accuracy of the information these resources provide.

The use of any information provided in this book is solely at your own risk.

1. Definition and Importance of Health Coaching

Health coaching is a patient-centered approach that involves facilitating individuals to cultivate healthier lifestyle choices and improve self-management of chronic health conditions. It encourages an individual to take an active role in their health journey by setting realistic health goals, developing strategies to achieve them, and navigating obstacles along the way.

The importance of health coaching cannot be overstated. With the rise in chronic diseases such as diabetes, heart disease, and obesity, the need for effective interventions to motivate and guide individuals to adopt healthier habits is paramount. Health coaching offers a promising solution by supporting individuals not only to manage their conditions but also to prevent disease through lifestyle changes.

2. Challenges in Health Coaching

Despite its significant potential, health coaching faces several challenges. One of the main challenges is non-compliance or non-adherence to medical advice and prescribed treatment plans. Many patients struggle to adhere to dietary, exercise, or medication regimens due to various factors, including lack of motivation, confusion, fear, or the perceived difficulty of making changes.

Another challenge is the one-size-fits-all approach that doesn't take into account the individual's unique needs, preferences, and circumstances. Health coaching requires tailoring strategies to each individual, which can be a time-consuming and complex process.

3. Introduction to Neuro-Linguistic Programming (NLP)

In order to achieve personal objectives, Neuro-Linguistic Programming (NLP), a psychological strategy, entails studying the techniques employed by successful people. It aims to understand how we think (neuro), how we communicate (linguistic), and how our patterns of behavior and emotion are organized (programming).

NLP encompasses a wide range of techniques, including establishing rapport, goal setting, identifying limiting beliefs, and modeling successful behaviors. The techniques used in NLP can help individuals to change their thought patterns, beliefs, and behaviors, leading to improved outcomes.

4. Rationale for Applying NLP in Health Coaching

Given the challenges in health coaching and the potential of NLP, it seems a natural progression to combine the two. Health coaching, by its very nature, seeks to motivate and support change in individuals, and NLP provides effective techniques for facilitating this change.

NLP's emphasis on understanding individual patterns and belief systems aligns with the personalized approach needed in health coaching. It provides strategies to overcome barriers to change and enhance motivation, which can significantly improve patient compliance and health outcomes.

Incorporating NLP into health coaching could address some of the limitations of traditional approaches, providing a more flexible, tailored, and potentially more effective strategy for supporting individuals in their health journey. By understanding and implementing NLP techniques, health coaches may better engage with their patients, enhance patient compliance, and ultimately, improve health outcomes.

1. History and Evolution of NLP

Neuro-Linguistic Programming (NLP) was first developed in the 1970s by Richard Bandler and John Grinder, a mathematician and a linguist respectively, at the University of California, Santa Cruz. They were interested in understanding how certain people excelled in their fields and if those skills could be replicated in others. Thus, NLP began as a process of modeling excellent communicators and therapists.

Through the years, NLP has evolved and incorporated insights from a range of disciplines, including cognitive psychology, gestalt therapy, and general semantics. It has expanded beyond the field of therapy and found applications in various areas such as business, sports, and education, and most relevantly to this book, health coaching.

2. Key Concepts of NLP

NLP revolves around several key concepts:

Modeling: The process of replicating the successful behaviors and beliefs of others.

Rapport: Building relationships based on trust and understanding.

Representational Systems: The idea that our perceptions of the world are represented in our mind through our senses.

Anchoring: The act of connecting an internal response to an outside trigger so that it can be easily and occasionally discreetly retrieved again.

Reframing: Changing the way one perceives an event and thus changing its meaning.

3. Misconceptions about NLP

Despite its potential, NLP has been surrounded by several misconceptions. Some see it as a manipulative tool, mainly because of its powerful influence over thoughts and behaviors.

However, like any tool, its ethical use depends on the practitioner. In health coaching, NLP can be used ethically to guide individuals towards healthier behaviors.

Another common misconception is that NLP is a quick fix for deep-seated issues. While NLP can bring about rapid changes, it should not replace comprehensive medical or psychological care when needed.

4. Clinical Evidence Supporting NLP

While NLP has been criticized for lacking empirical support, a growing body of research suggests that NLP techniques can have positive effects. Studies have shown that NLP can be effective in reducing stress, improving mood, enhancing communication skills, and promoting behavior change.

In the realm of health coaching, there's increasing interest in harnessing NLP's power to enhance patient compliance and improve health outcomes. Several studies indicate that NLP can contribute to improved self-management of chronic diseases, increased physical activity, and healthier dietary habits.

However, more research is needed to fully understand the mechanisms of NLP and the most effective ways to apply it in the field of health coaching. As the body of evidence grows, so too will the understanding and application of NLP within this important realm of healthcare.

1. Understanding the Linguistic Aspect of NLP in Health Coaching

The linguistic aspect of NLP concerns how we use language to shape our thoughts, emotions, and behaviors. For health coaches, understanding a patient's language patterns can provide insight into their mental representations of health and illness.

For example, a patient might say, "I can't stop eating sweets." The use of "can't" suggests a belief of impossibility. A health coach trained in NLP would pick up on this language pattern and might ask, "What would happen if you could?" This could help the patient explore their beliefs about their ability to change.

2. Anchoring and Its Application in Health Behaviour Change

Anchoring involves associating a specific emotional state or physical sensation with a particular stimulus. For instance, a health coach might help a patient anchor the feeling of motivation to a visual cue, such as a motivational poster.

Once the anchor is set, the patient can use the visual cue to access the desired state (motivation) when needed, like before a workout. This can help overcome barriers to exercise, one of the common challenges in lifestyle change.

3. Reframing Perspectives for Healthier Choices

Reframing is a powerful NLP technique that involves changing the meaning of an experience by viewing it from a different perspective. For instance, a patient might view exercise as a chore. A health coach could reframe this perspective by helping the patient see exercise as an opportunity for self-care or a way to increase energy levels.

By reframing the meaning of exercise, the health coach can help the patient shift their attitude towards a healthier choice, thus promoting behavior change.

4. Utilization of Metaphors for Change

NLP makes extensive use of metaphors to facilitate change. Metaphors can bypass resistance and speak directly to the unconscious mind.

For instance, a health coach might use the metaphor of a journey for a patient's path to better health. By envisioning health as a journey, the patient may better understand that progress requires time and effort, and that there may be setbacks along the way. This can help foster patience, persistence, and resilience.

5. The Milton Model and Its Application in Health Coaching

The Milton Model, named after the renowned hypnotherapist Milton Erickson, is a set of linguistic patterns designed to guide someone into a hypnotic state, allowing them to access and utilize their unconscious resources.

In health coaching, the Milton Model can be used to help patients tap into their internal resources for change. For example, a health coach might say, "You might not yet know how capable you are of making these healthy changes, just as you might not yet realize all the ways these changes will improve your life."

This vague language allows patients to fill in the blanks with their own meanings, thus enhancing their motivation and commitment to change.

1. The Role of NLP in Influencing Patient Compliance

Patient compliance, the degree to which a patient correctly follows medical advice, is a critical factor in health outcomes. The use of NLP techniques can significantly influence patient compliance by addressing underlying beliefs and emotions that impact health behaviors.

For instance, using techniques such as reframing or anchoring, a health coach can help a patient shift their perception of a prescribed treatment from being a burden to being a necessary step toward better health. Moreover, through modeling, a coach can guide patients to emulate the behaviors of individuals who successfully adhere to similar treatment plans.

2. <u>Hypothetical</u> Case Studies: Successful Application of NLP in Enhancing Patient Compliance

Consider the case of a 58-year-old diabetic patient who struggled with medication adherence due to a belief that her medication was a sign of weakness. A health coach using NLP reframed this perspective by associating medication adherence with strength - the strength to take control of her health and life. Consequently, the patient's medication adherence improved dramatically, leading to better control of her diabetes.

In another hypothetical case, a young man with hypertension had poor compliance with his exercise regimen. A health coach used the NLP technique of anchoring to associate the state of feeling energized and positive with the act of exercise. This resulted in improved exercise compliance, contributing to better management of his hypertension.

3. Strategies for Implementing NLP to Improve Compliance

To effectively implement NLP in improving patient compliance, health coaches can consider the following strategies:

Individualized Approach: Tailor the use of NLP techniques to each patient's unique needs, preferences, and circumstances. Rapport Building: Establish a strong rapport with patients to enhance trust and openness, making NLP interventions more effective.

Empowerment: Use NLP to help patients uncover their internal resources and strengths, which can boost their self-efficacy and motivation to adhere to treatment plans.

Continuous Learning: As a health coach, constantly upgrade your knowledge and skills in NLP and stay updated on the latest research.

The application of NLP techniques in health coaching requires skilled use and ethical consideration. Done correctly, it holds considerable promise in enhancing patient compliance and, consequently, improving health outcomes.

1. NLP Techniques to Boost Patient Confidence and Self-Efficacy

Confidence and self-efficacy play a crucial role in managing health and lifestyle changes. NLP can provide techniques to enhance these attributes. For instance, the 'Circle of Excellence' is a popular NLP technique to boost confidence. This involves having the patient imagine a circle on the ground filled with all the resources they need, such as courage, determination, and optimism. The patient steps into the circle, embodying these qualities, effectively anchoring them for future use.

2. Using NLP to Manage Pain and Chronic Health Conditions

NLP offers several techniques that can assist patients in managing pain and chronic health conditions. For example, the technique of 'dissociation' helps patients manage pain by encouraging them to separate themselves from their discomfort. They could visualize their pain as an image or color and then mentally manipulate that image to lessen the pain's intensity.

For chronic conditions like diabetes, NLP can be used to anchor positive feelings to the necessary self-care activities, such as checking blood sugar levels or adhering to a specific diet, making these activities more manageable and less stressful.

3. Strategies for Integrating NLP into the Patient Care Journey

To integrate NLP effectively into the patient care journey, health coaches can:

Begin with a thorough assessment of the patient's beliefs, language patterns, and behavioral strategies.

Collaboratively set realistic and achievable health goals using NLP's well-formed outcomes criteria.

Use NLP techniques, such as anchoring and reframing, throughout the patient care journey to support behavior change.

Regularly review and revise the plan according to the patient's progress, using NLP techniques to overcome new obstacles or resistance.

4. Hypothetical Case Studies: Improvements in Health Outcomes Through NLP

Consider a patient with obesity struggling with adhering to a diet plan. The patient may believe they cannot resist the temptation of unhealthy foods. A health coach could use NLP reframing techniques to help the patient view these foods not as tempting indulgences but as obstacles to their health and well-being. By changing the patient's perception, the coach can help the patient make healthier food choices, leading to weight loss and improved health outcomes.

In another hypothetical case, a patient suffering from chronic migraines could use the dissociation technique to manage their pain better. By visualizing their pain as an object and then altering that object's size, color, or distance, the patient can effectively reduce the perceived intensity of the pain.

These hypothetical cases illustrate the potential of NLP to improve health outcomes by influencing perceptions, emotions, and behaviors related to health and disease.

1. Addressing NLP Skepticism

NLP has faced criticism due to a lack of large-scale, high-quality scientific studies to back its effectiveness, leading to skepticism among some medical professionals. Health coaches can address this skepticism by staying informed about the latest research in NLP, participating in ongoing education, and openly discussing NLP's potential benefits and limitations with patients and other healthcare providers.

2. Training Health Coaches in NLP

While there are many NLP training programs available, they vary widely in depth, duration, and quality. Thus, finding a reputable program that provides comprehensive, evidence-based training in NLP can be a challenge. Health coaches interested in NLP should carefully evaluate potential programs, looking for those that incorporate scientific evidence, include practical training, and are taught by experienced and credentialed professionals.

3. Ethical Considerations in Using NLP

As with any tool that can influence behavior and perception, NLP must be used ethically. Coaches should always respect patients' autonomy and use NLP techniques to empower patients rather than manipulate them. Transparency about the use of NLP and its purpose is essential. Furthermore, NLP should not be used as a substitute for necessary medical care or mental health support.

4. Future Research in NLP and Health Coaching

While there's growing evidence for NLP's effectiveness in health coaching, more research is needed. Future research could explore how different NLP techniques affect various health outcomes, identify which patients might benefit most from NLP, and determine the most effective ways to integrate NLP into health coaching.

Furthermore, research should aim to understand the mechanisms through which NLP influences behavior and health outcomes. Understanding these mechanisms can help refine NLP techniques and make them more effective in promoting health and wellbeing.

The continued exploration of NLP's potential in health coaching holds promise for overcoming existing barriers and leveraging this powerful tool to improve patient compliance and health outcomes.

1. Summarizing the Impact of NLP in Health Coaching

Neuro-Linguistic Programming, with its rich array of techniques for influencing thoughts, emotions, and behaviors, offers a powerful toolset for health coaching. From enhancing patient compliance to improving health outcomes, NLP can substantially impact patients' lives. The linguistic, sensory, and cognitive strategies that NLP provides can guide patients in reframing limiting beliefs, establishing healthy behaviors, managing chronic conditions, and achieving their health goals.

2. Implications for Health Coaches and Patients

For health coaches, mastering NLP can amplify their impact on patients. It allows coaches to decipher patients' cognitive and linguistic patterns, helping to tailor interventions to individual needs. For patients, engaging with a health coach skilled in NLP can offer a new lens to view their health and an empowering path to behavior change.

However, both coaches and patients need to approach NLP with openness, critical thinking, and an understanding of its limitations. NLP is not a cure-all but a valuable addition to the holistic toolbox of health coaching.

3. Future Directions for NLP in Health Coaching

As more research is conducted, we can expect deeper insights into the most effective uses of NLP in health coaching. Future directions might include the development of standardized NLP training programs for health coaches, integration of NLP with other behavioral interventions, and the creation of evidence-based NLP protocols for specific health issues.

4. Final Thoughts and Encouragements for Health Coaches

As a health coach, your role is to guide, support, and empower your patients. Integrating NLP into your practice could enhance your ability to fulfill this role. It's important to approach NLP with a learner's mindset, continually seeking to expand your knowledge and skills.

Remember, the goal is not just to apply NLP techniques, but to use them in a way that truly honors and respects each patient's unique journey towards health and well-being. This integration of expertise, empathy, and ethical practice is what can truly elevate your impact as a health coach.

Rex Morton is a renowned author and researcher in the United Kingdom with a passionate interest in the human mind, specifically in Cognitive Behavioural Therapy (CBT) and Neuro-Linguistic Programming (NLP).

Morton has spent a considerable portion of his professional life diving deep into the theories and principles that form the backbone of these two compelling fields. His fascination with NLP led him to complete an extensive certification program, solidifying his understanding of this innovative approach to understanding human behaviour.

Although Morton does not have clinical experience, his intense curiosity and dedication to studying these subjects have made him a respected figure in the field. He has thoroughly researched the integration of NLP techniques into CBT, offering fresh perspectives and insights into how these two methodologies can complement each other to enhance understanding of human cognition and behaviour.

As an author, Morton has successfully communicated his knowledge and passion to a broader audience, making complex psychological theories accessible to professionals and interested laypersons. His writing is characterized by a clear, engaging style and a focus on the practical application of theories, making them relevant to everyday life.

In his personal life, Morton is an ardent lover of the natural world, often spending his free time exploring the British countryside. His passion for landscape photography allows him to capture and share the beauty of these excursions. Despite his accomplishments, Morton is known for his humility and eagerness to continue learning. His work continues to inspire those interested in the intricate workings of the human mind and the exciting possibilities presented by the integration of NLP and CBT.

If you've found the content of this book enlightening and wish to continue your journey of understanding the human mind, I warmly invite you to visit my website at www.rexmorton.com. The website serves as a hub of knowledge where I share my latest findings, thoughts, and insights on the integration of NLP and CBT.

I also encourage you to subscribe to the newsletter available on the website. By subscribing, you'll receive regular updates on a range of topics, from detailed discussions on specific NLP techniques and their application in CBT, to the latest research in the field.

The newsletter is also the first place I'll share news of upcoming releases. Whether it's the announcement of a new book, the launch of an online course, newsletter subscribers will be the first to know. This is a great opportunity to continue learning directly from me, deepening your understanding of NLP and CBT, and enhancing your skills in applying these techniques in your own life or professional practice.

I'm looking forward to sharing this journey with you.